# JAMES

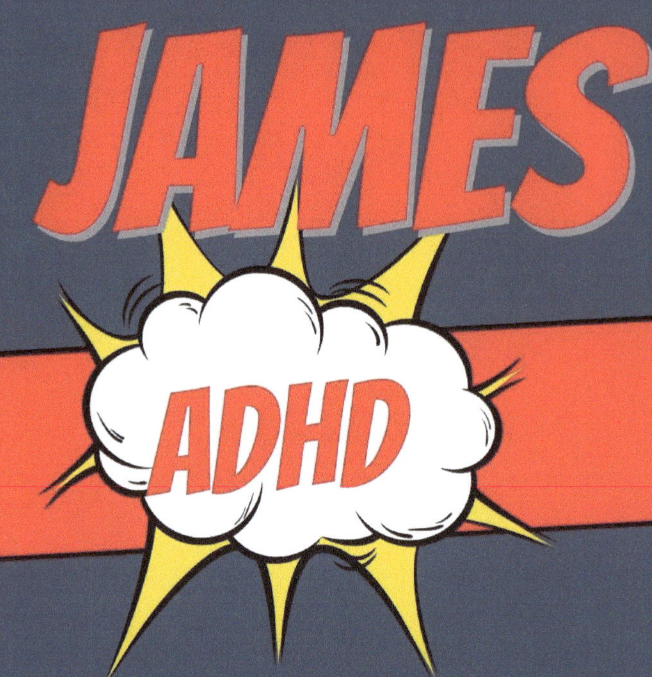


## BY J.J. MCBRIDGE

## TAKES A TRIP AROUND THE SOLAR SYSTEM!

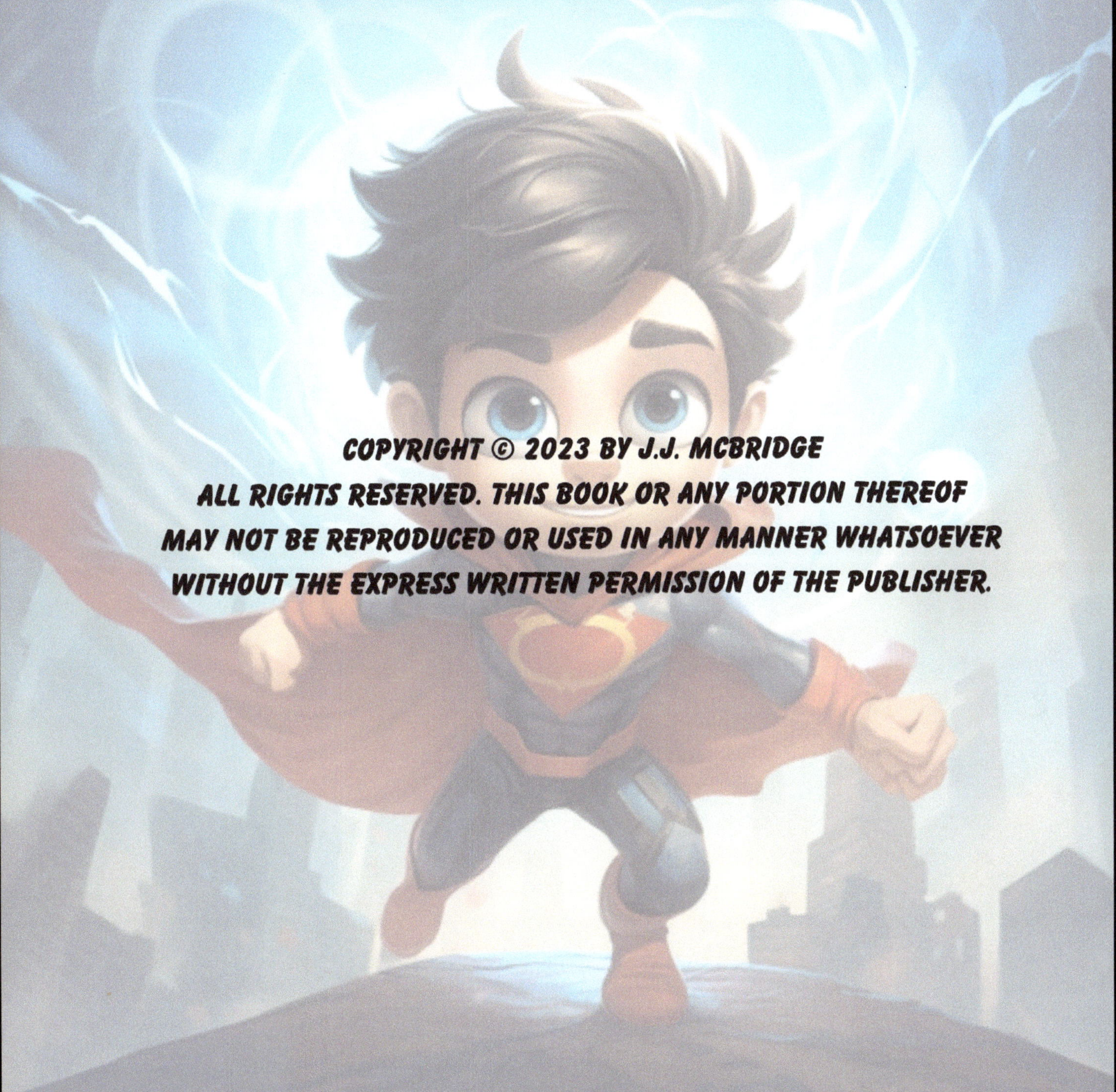

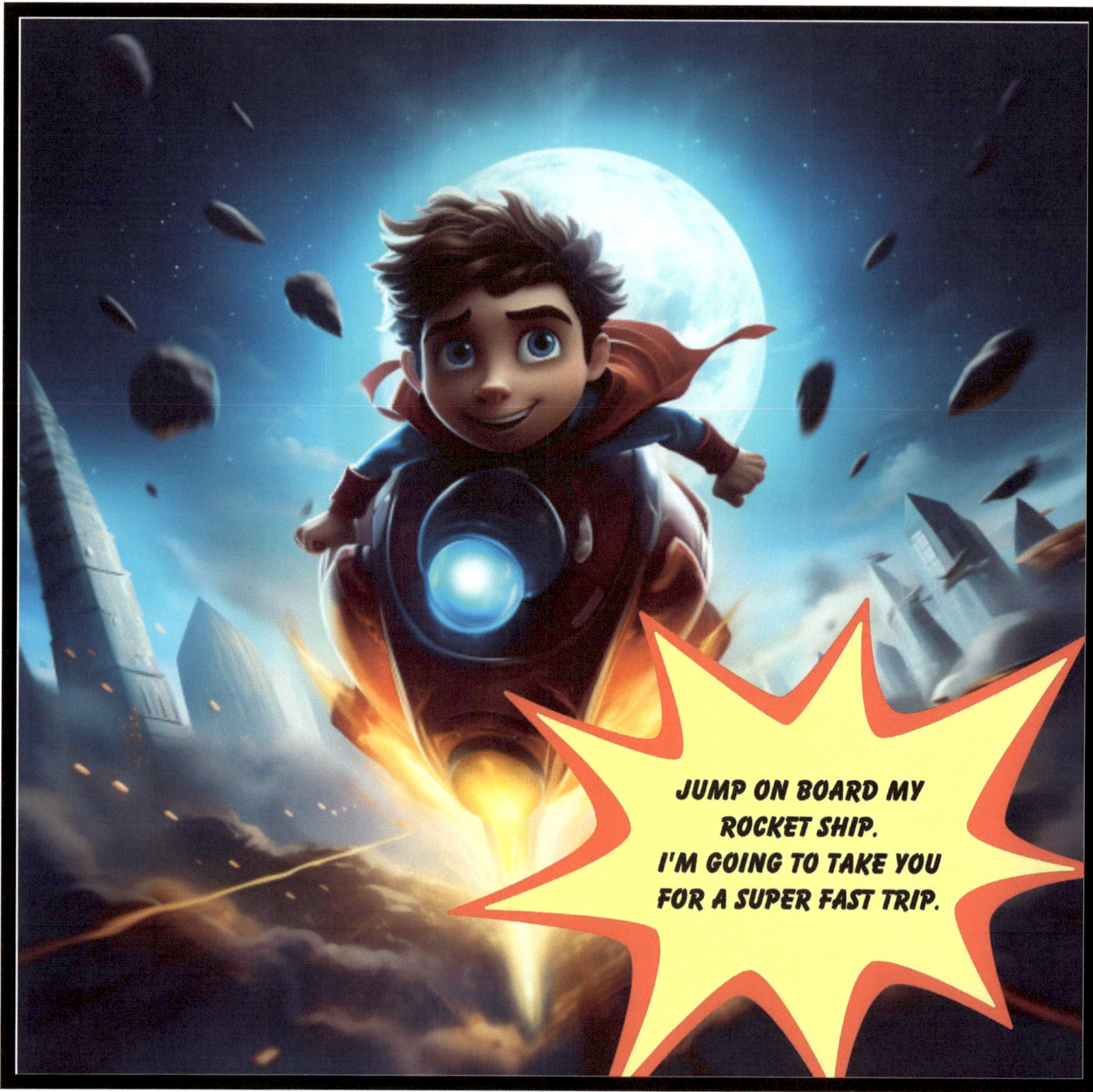

JUMP ON BOARD MY ROCKET SHIP.
I'M GOING TO TAKE YOU FOR A SUPER FAST TRIP.

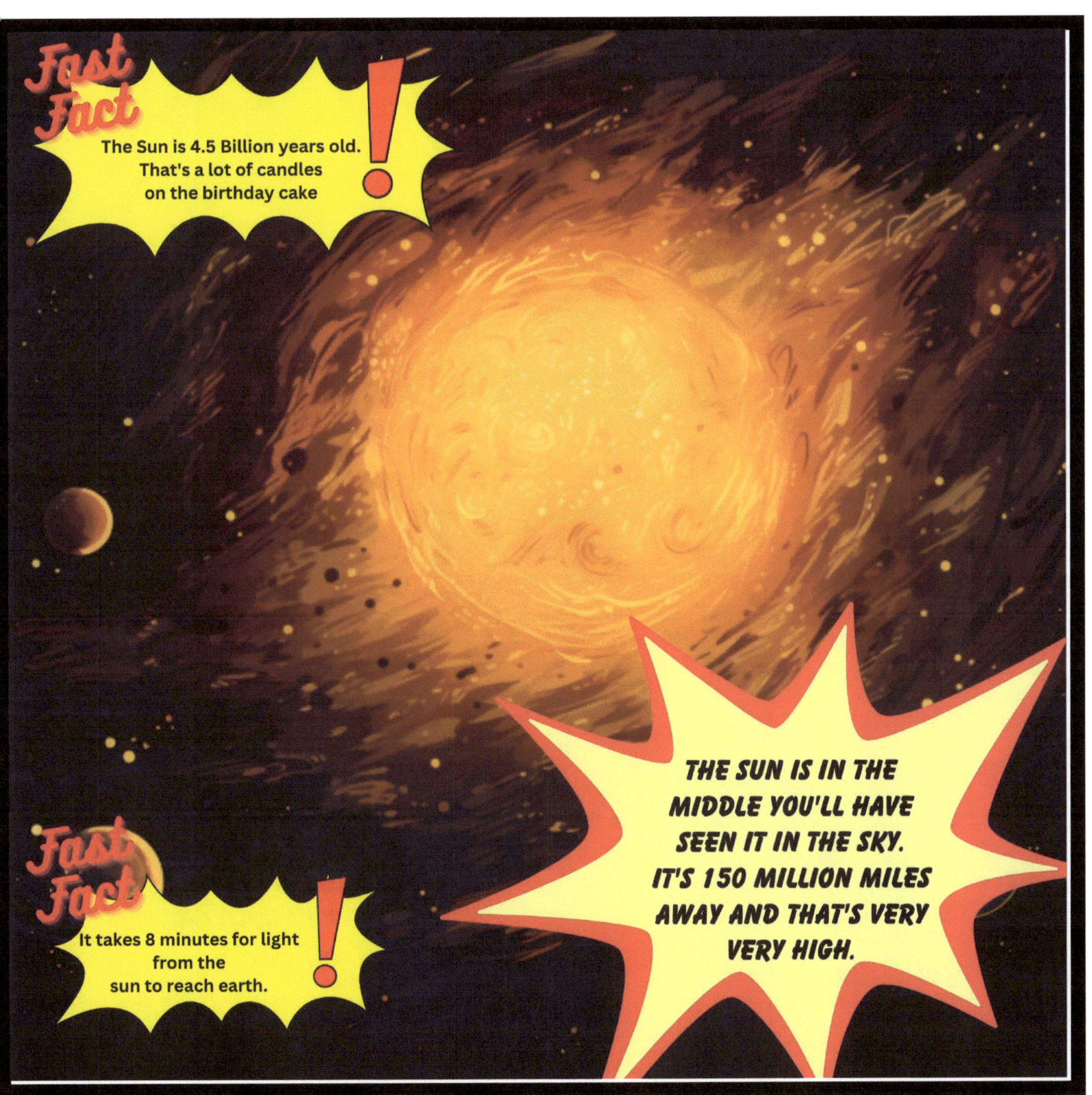

Fast Fact
The Sun is 4.5 Billion years old. That's a lot of candles on the birthday cake
Fast Fact
It takes 8 minutes for light from the sun to reach earth.
THE SUN IS IN THE MIDDLE YOU'LL HAVE SEEN IT IN THE SKY. IT'S 150 MILLION MILES AWAY AND THAT'S VERY VERY HIGH.

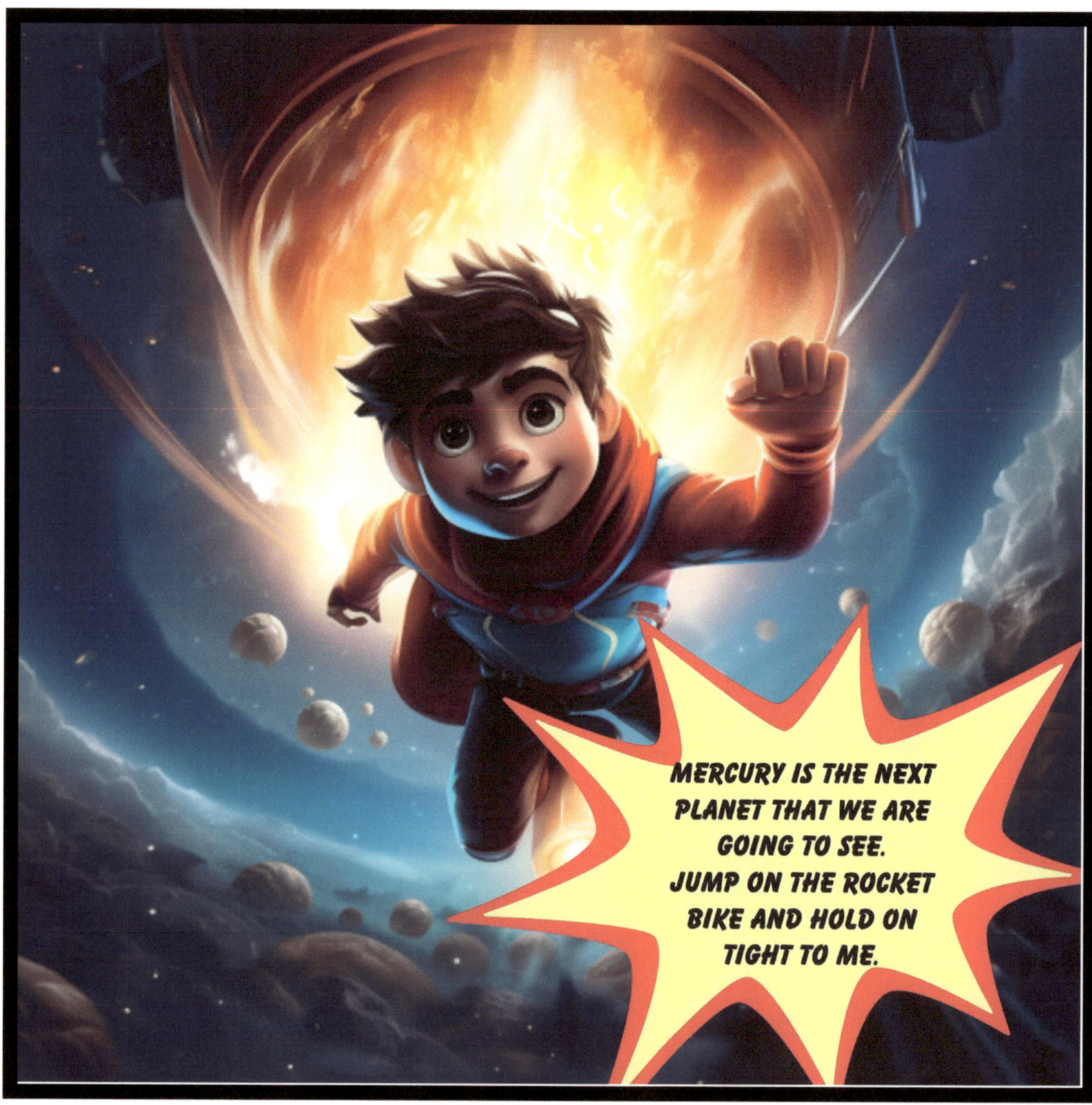
MERCURY IS THE NEXT PLANET THAT WE ARE GOING TO SEE. JUMP ON THE ROCKET BIKE AND HOLD ON TIGHT TO ME.

# MERCURY

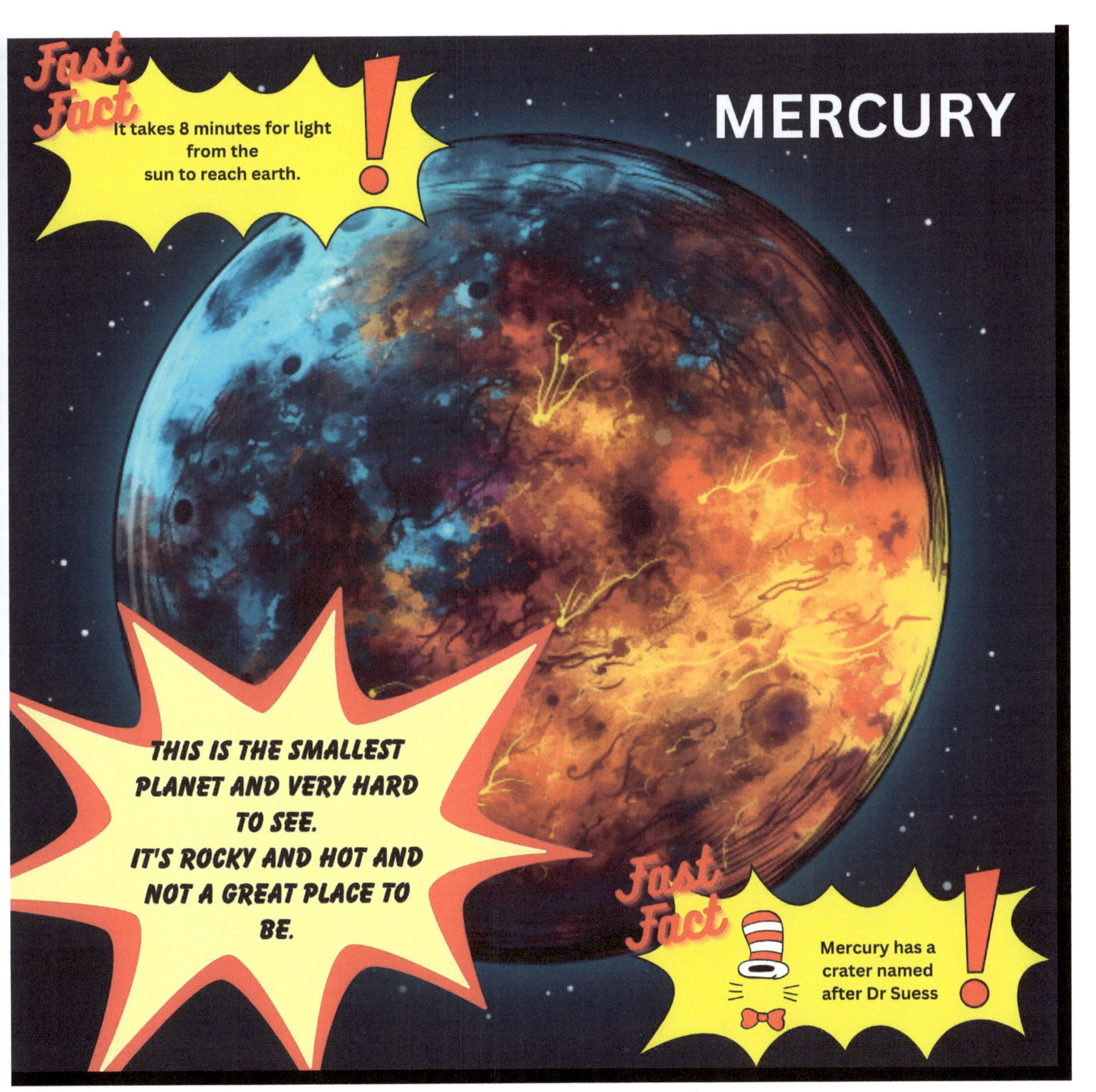

Fast Fact
It takes 8 minutes for light from the sun to reach earth.
!
THIS IS THE SMALLEST PLANET AND VERY HARD TO SEE.
IT'S ROCKY AND HOT AND NOT A GREAT PLACE TO BE.
Fast Fact
Mercury has a crater named after Dr Suess
!

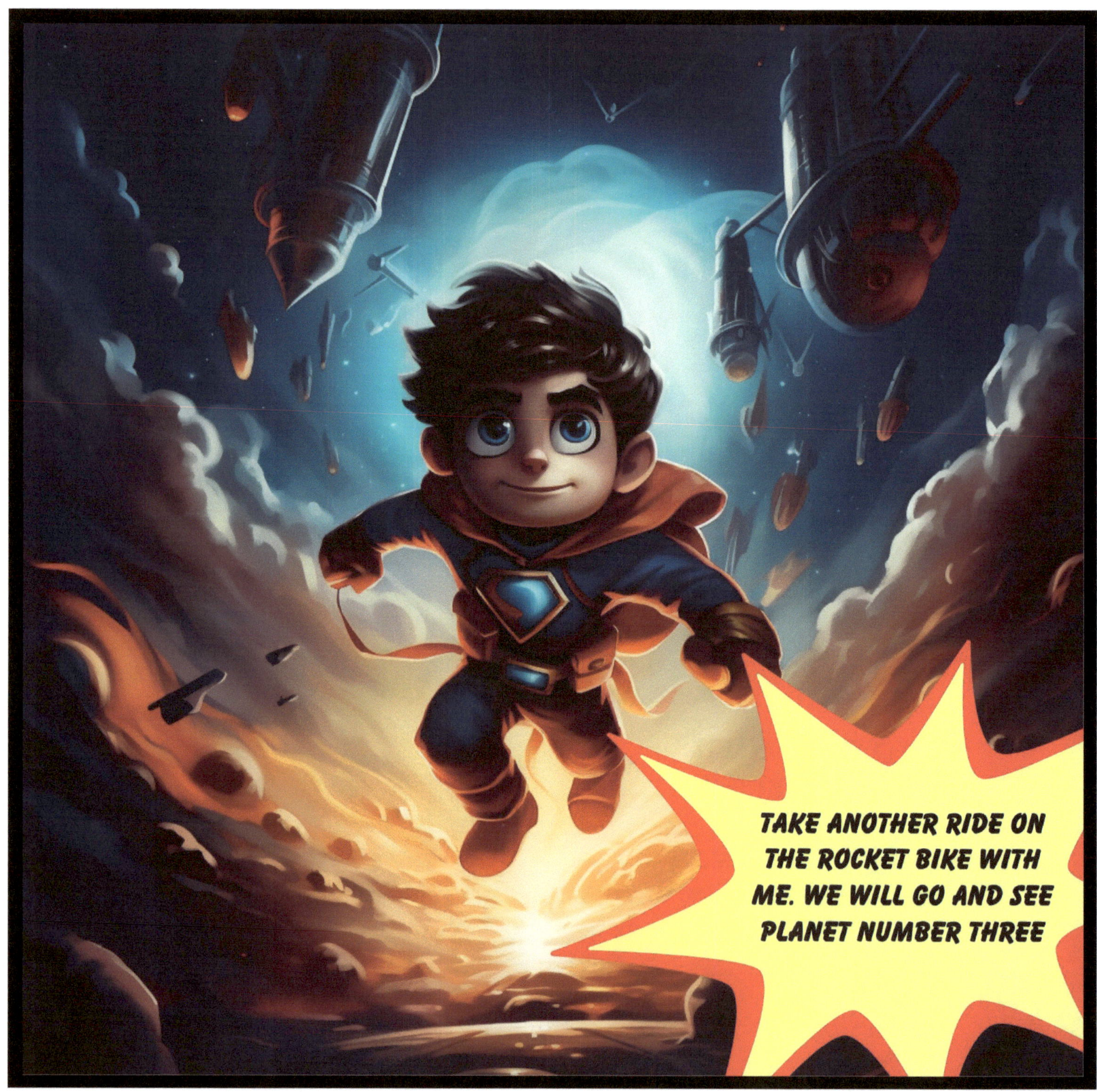

TAKE ANOTHER RIDE ON THE ROCKET BIKE WITH ME. WE WILL GO AND SEE PLANET NUMBER THREE

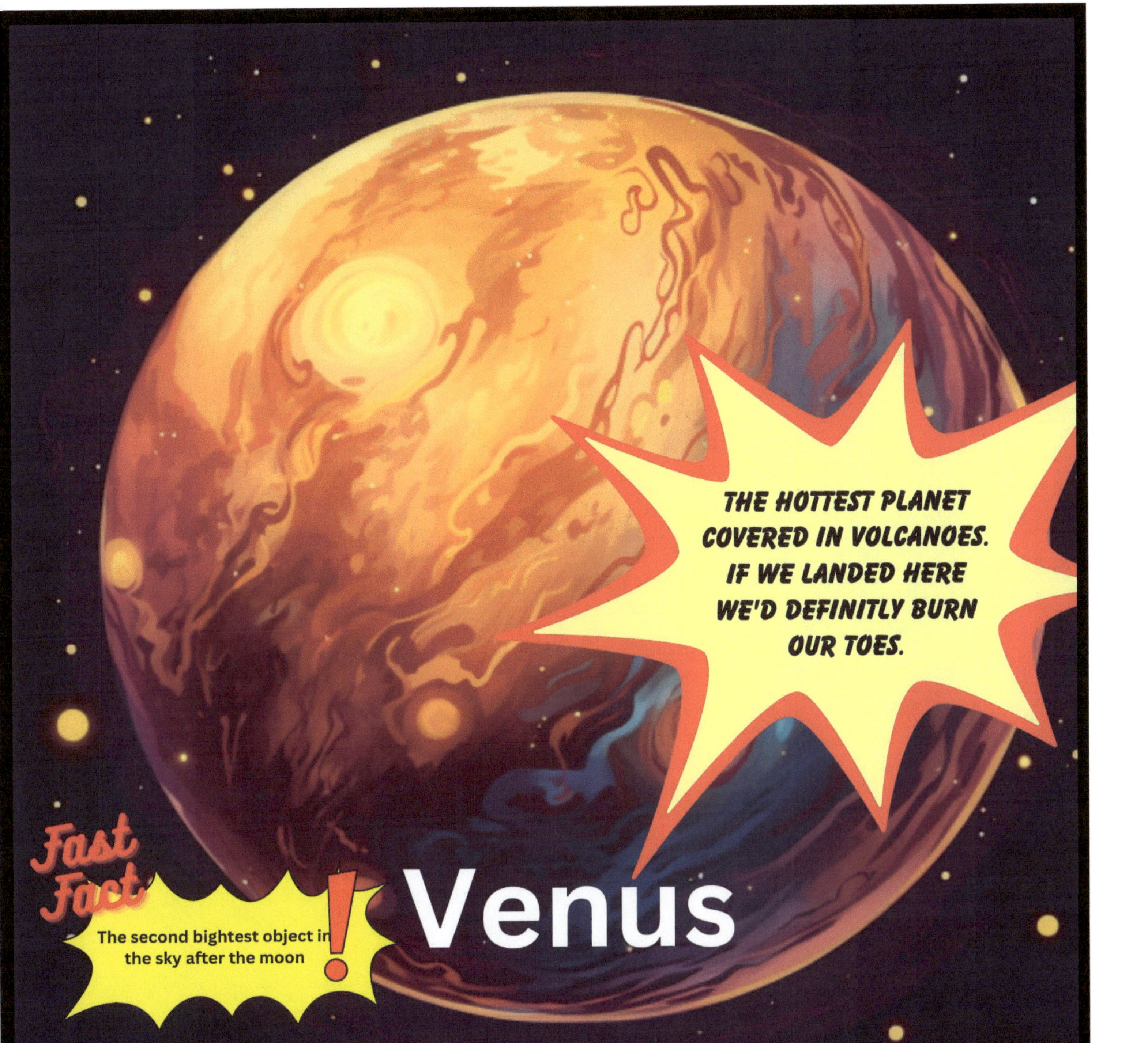

THE HOTTEST PLANET COVERED IN VOLCANOES. IF WE LANDED HERE WE'D DEFINITLY BURN OUR TOES.
Fast Fact
The second bightest object in the sky after the moon
Venus

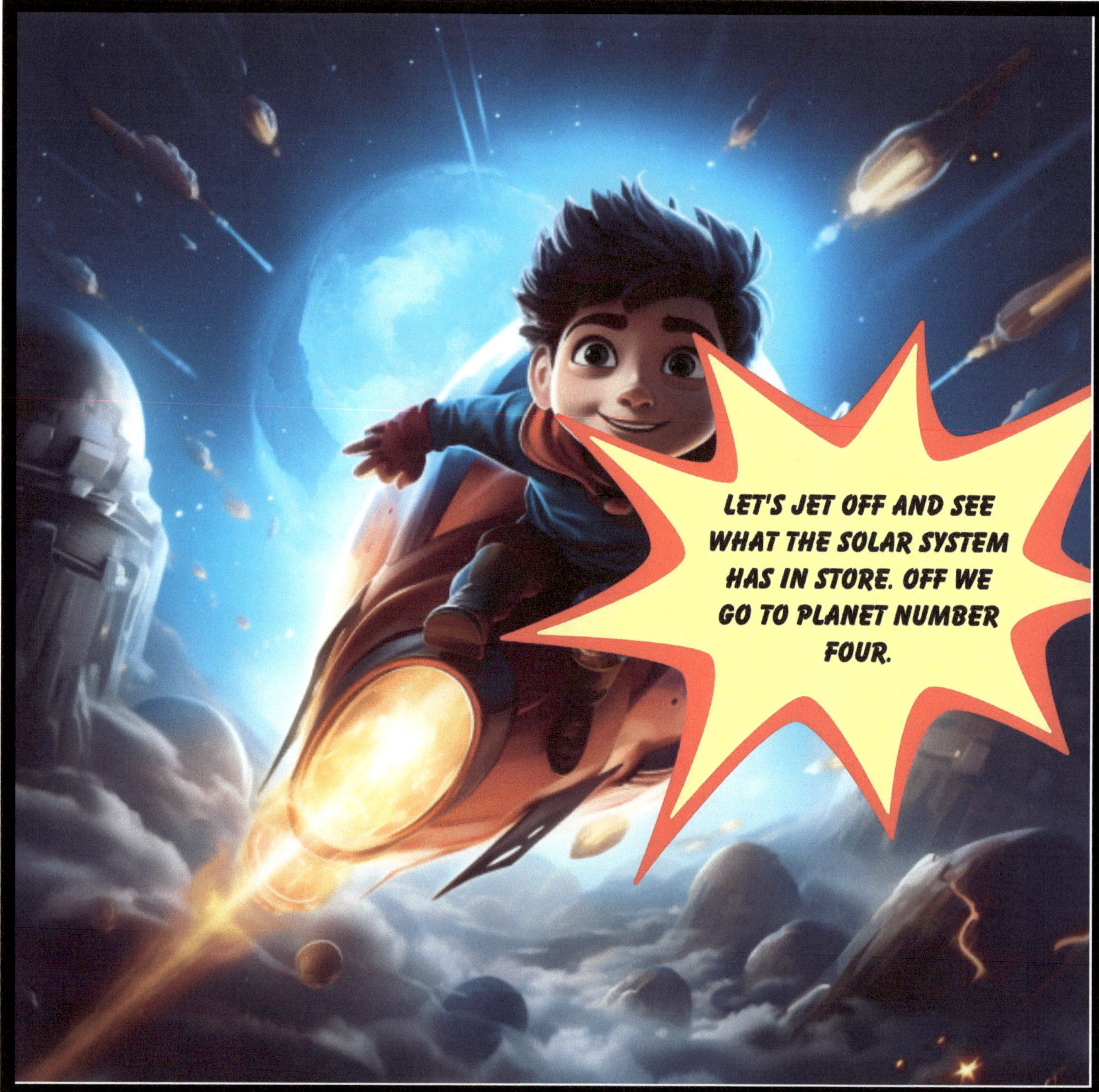

LET'S JET OFF AND SEE WHAT THE SOLAR SYSTEM HAS IN STORE. OFF WE GO TO PLANET NUMBER FOUR.

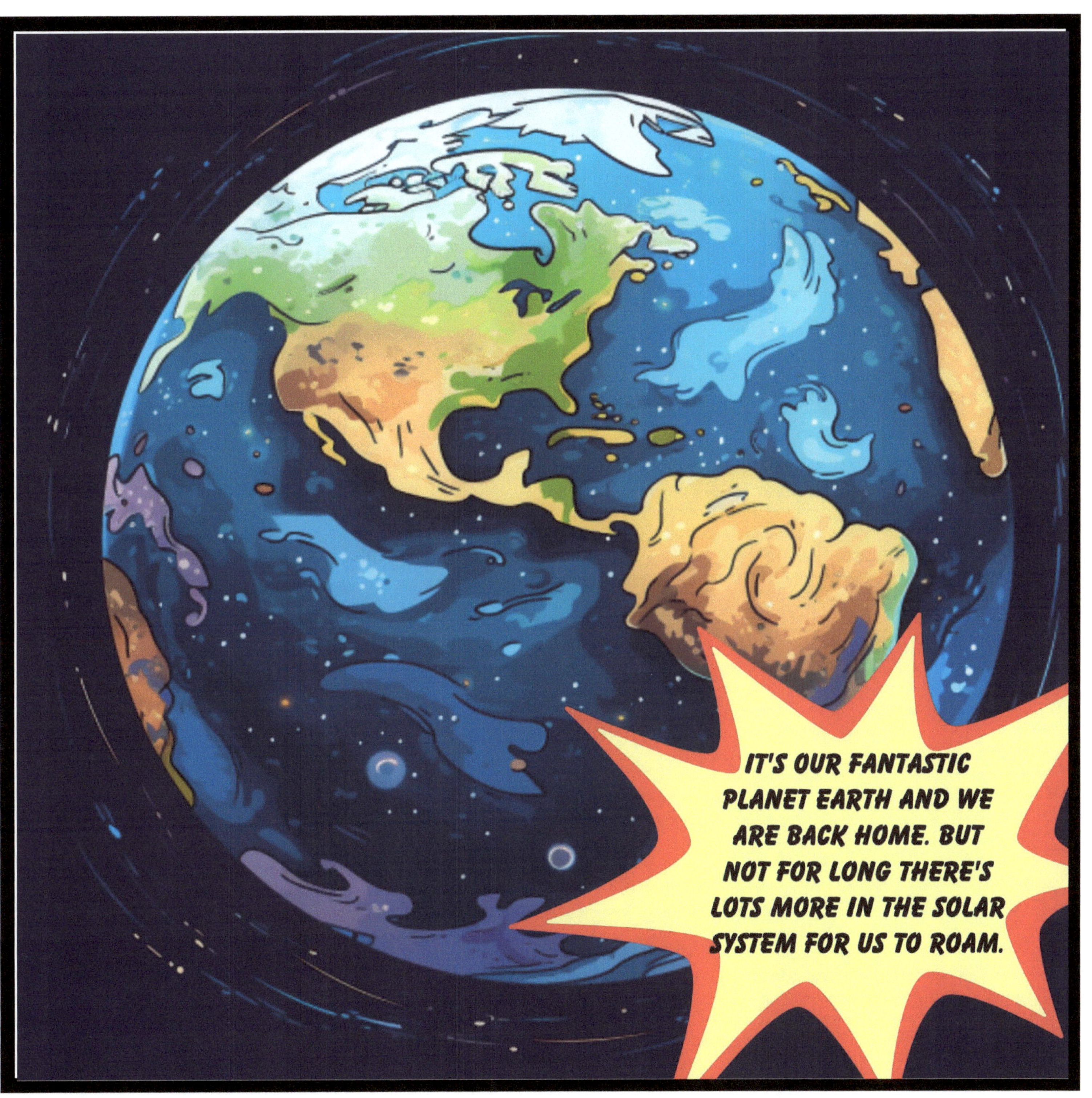
IT'S OUR FANTASTIC PLANET EARTH AND WE ARE BACK HOME. BUT NOT FOR LONG THERE'S LOTS MORE IN THE SOLAR SYSTEM FOR US TO ROAM.

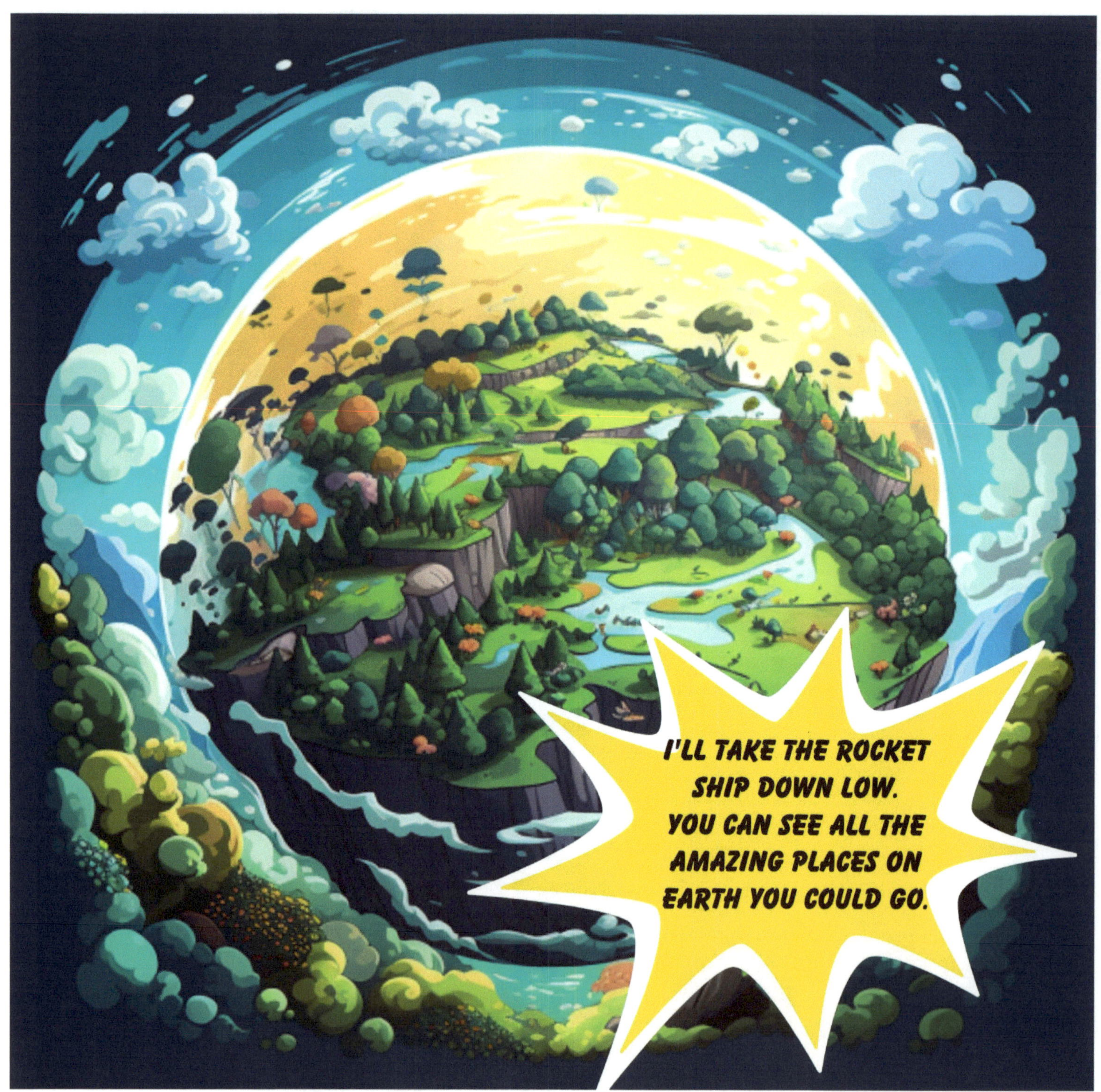
I'LL TAKE THE ROCKET SHIP DOWN LOW. YOU CAN SEE ALL THE AMAZING PLACES ON EARTH YOU COULD GO.

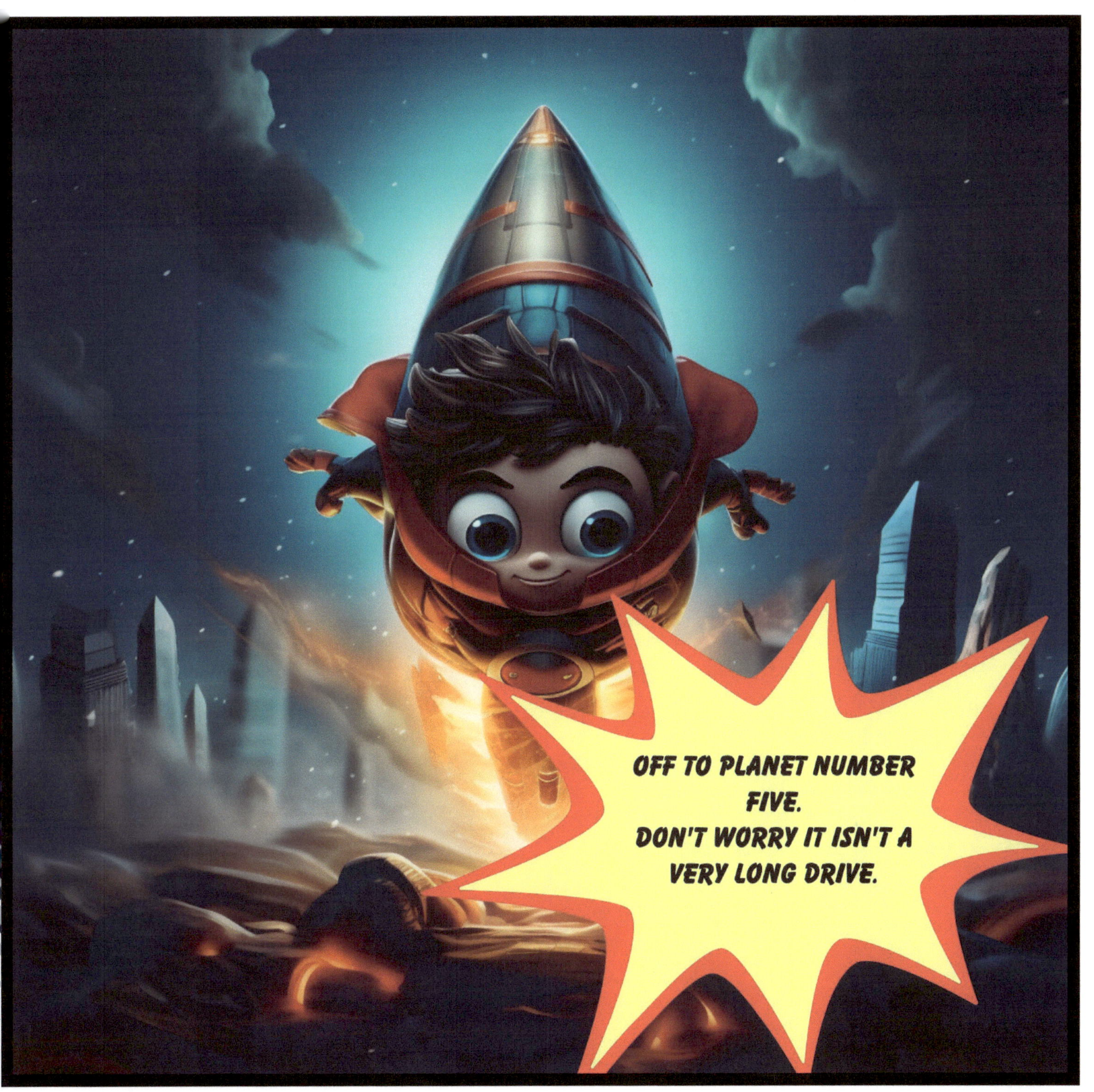

OFF TO PLANET NUMBER
FIVE.
DON'T WORRY IT ISN'T A
VERY LONG DRIVE.

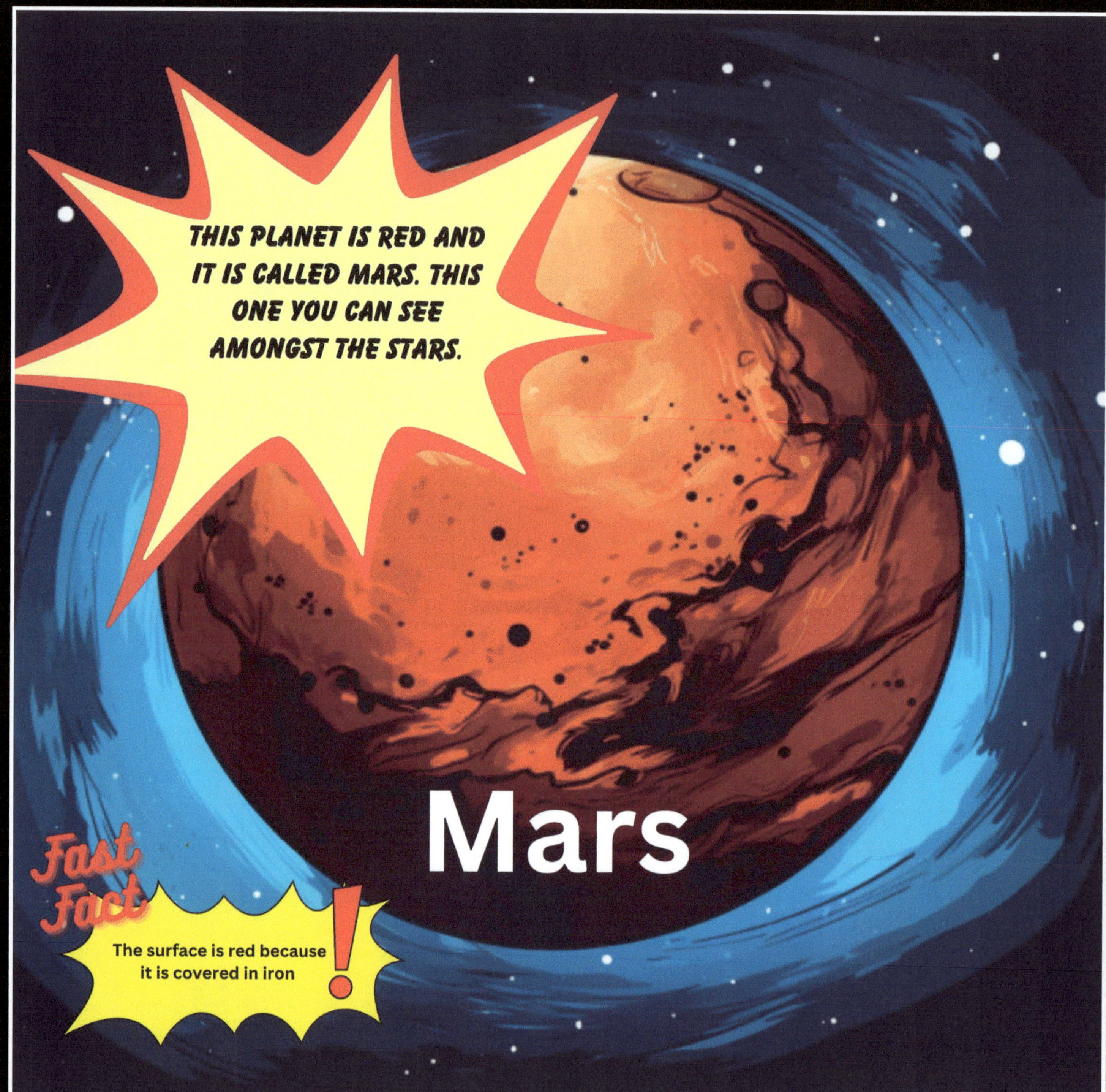

THIS PLANET IS RED AND IT IS CALLED MARS. THIS ONE YOU CAN SEE AMONGST THE STARS.
Mars
Fast Fact
The surface is red because it is covered in iron !

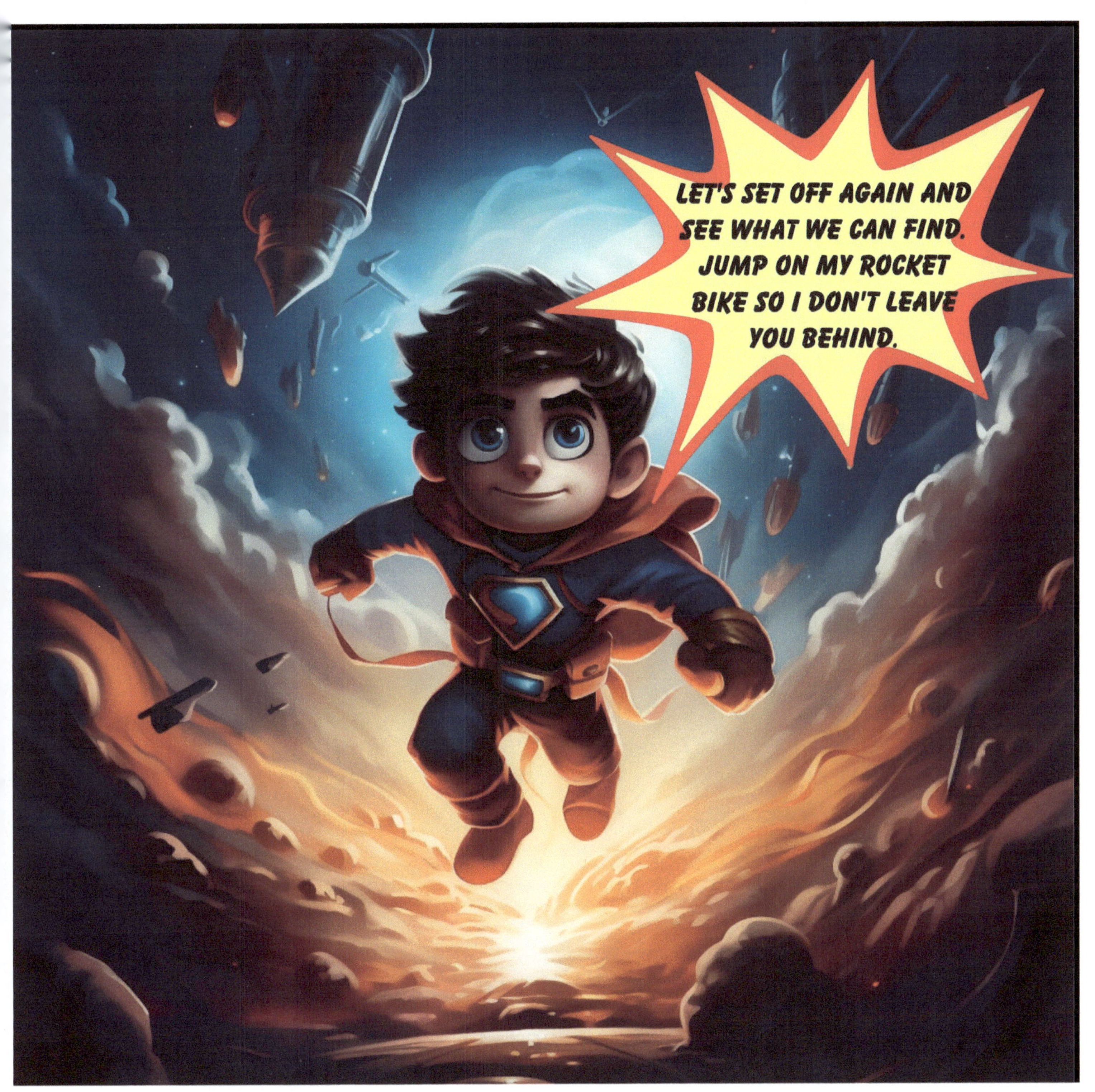

LET'S SET OFF AGAIN AND SEE WHAT WE CAN FIND. JUMP ON MY ROCKET BIKE SO I DON'T LEAVE YOU BEHIND.

# Jupitor

Fast Fact
Jupitor is the largest planet in the solar system
JUPITOR IS THE BIGGEST PLANET IN THE SKY. IT IS A GAS GIANT YOU CAN SEE THE SWIRLING STORMS AS WE FLY BY.

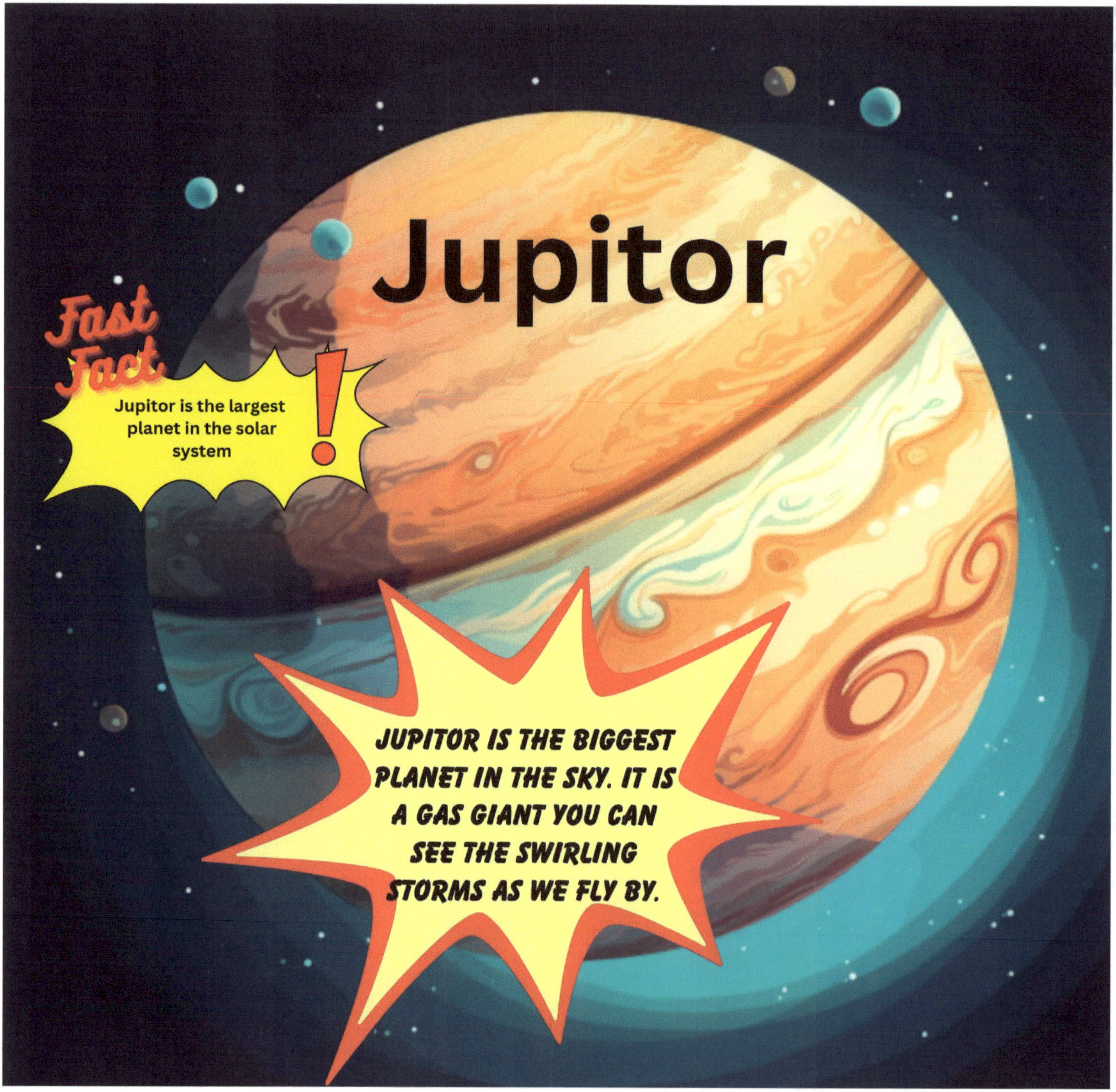

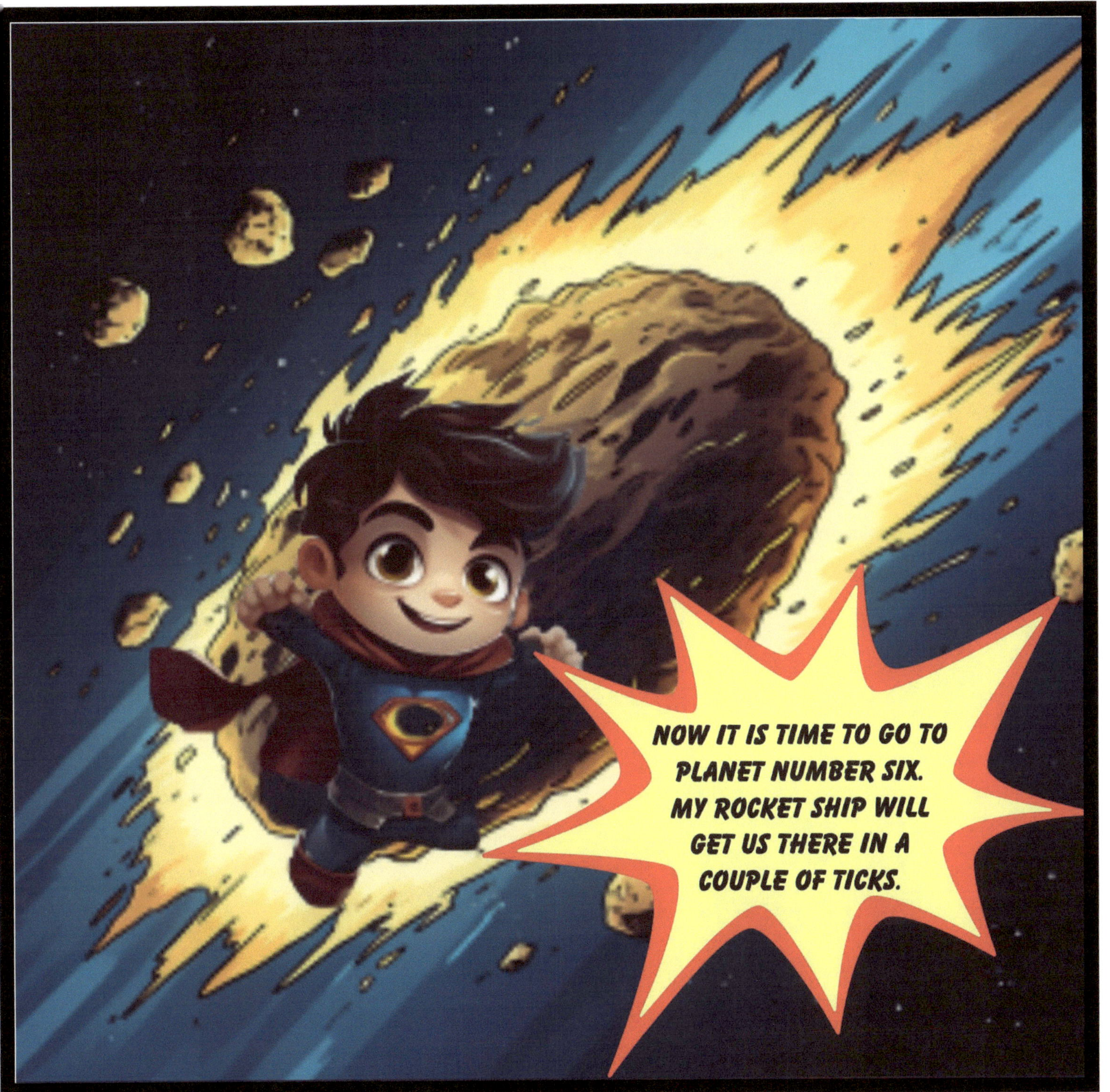

NOW IT IS TIME TO GO TO
PLANET NUMBER SIX.
MY ROCKET SHIP WILL
GET US THERE IN A
COUPLE OF TICKS.

# Saturn

FAST
FACT
Jupitor is the largest planet in the solar system
!
SATURN IS SO PRETTY WITH IT'S FAMOUS RINGS BUT IT'S ONLY MADE OF GAS.
SO WE CAN'T STOP HERE WE WILL JUST HAVE TO FLY RIGHT PAST.

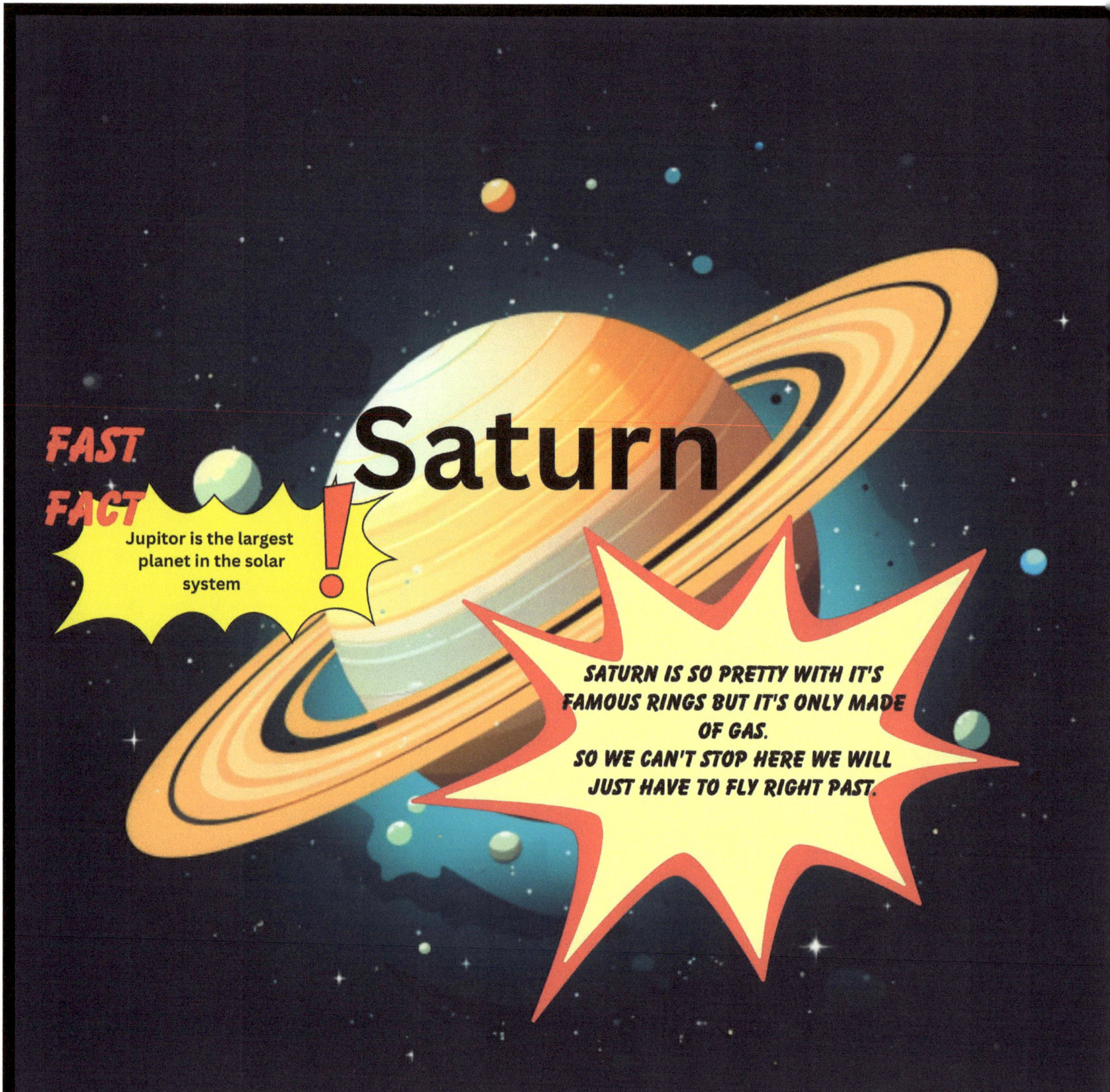

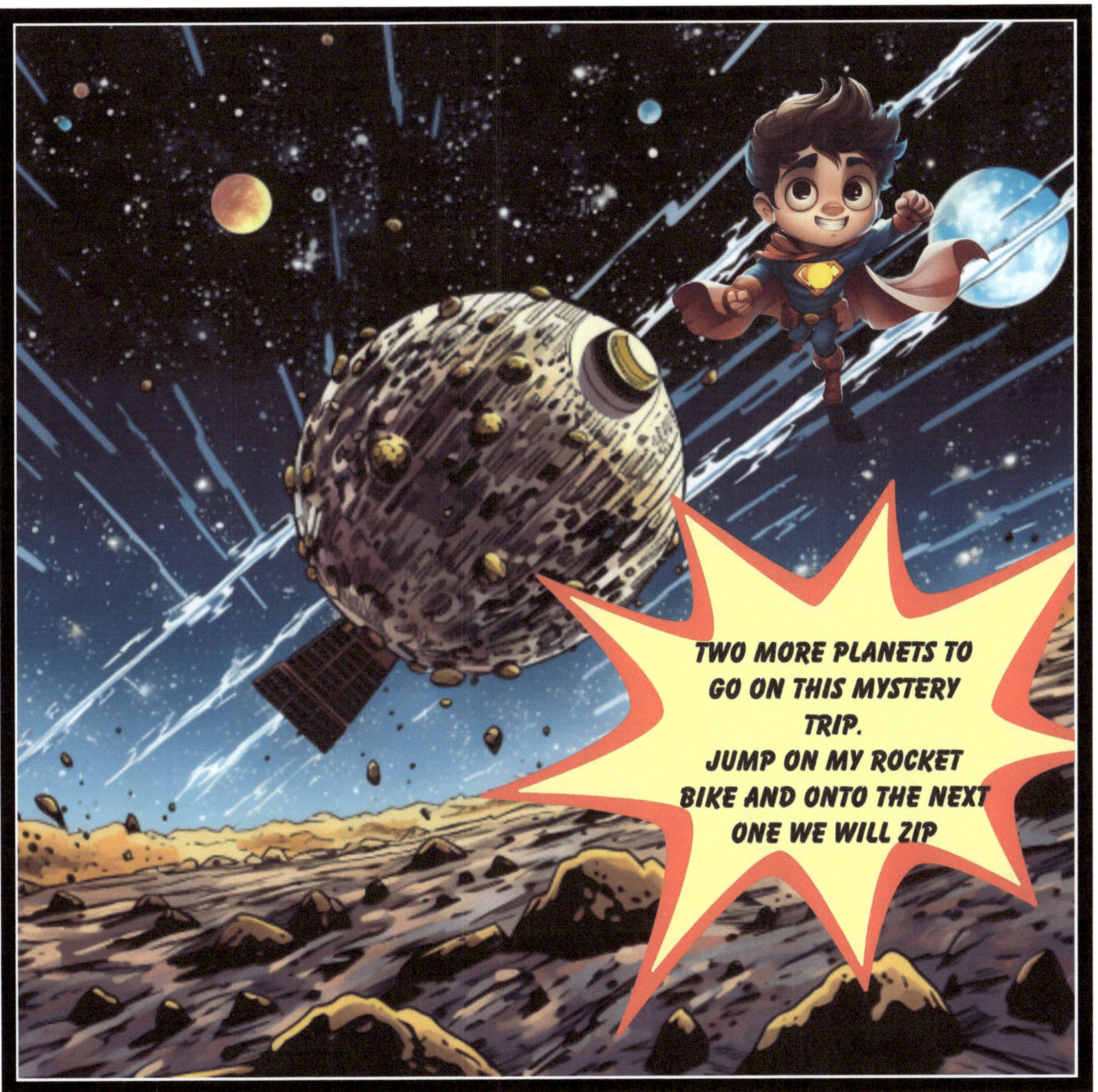

TWO MORE PLANETS TO GO ON THIS MYSTERY TRIP.
JUMP ON MY ROCKET BIKE AND ONTO THE NEXT ONE WE WILL ZIP

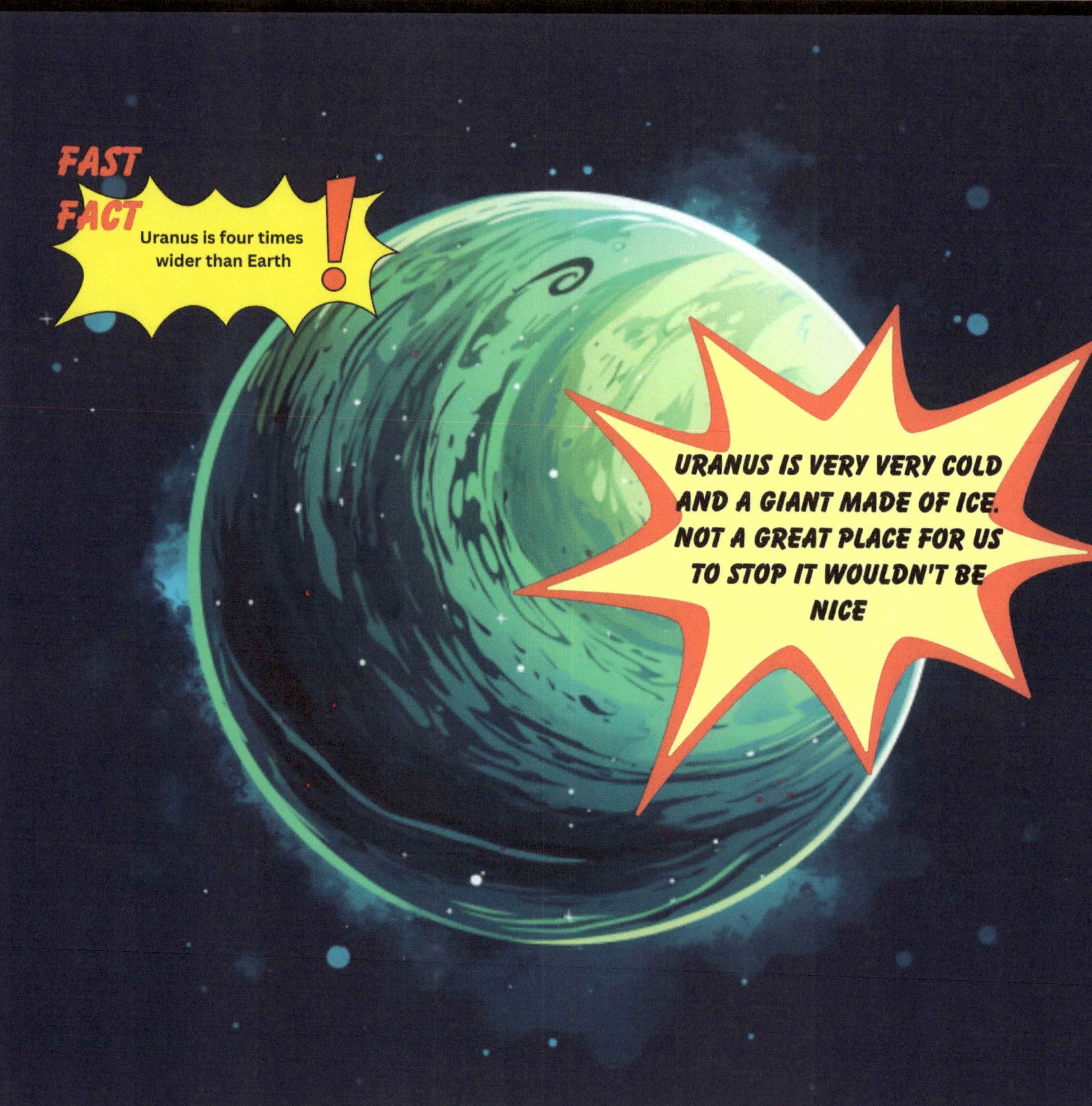

FAST FACT
Uranus is four times wider than Earth
!
URANUS IS VERY VERY COLD AND A GIANT MADE OF ICE. NOT A GREAT PLACE FOR US TO STOP IT WOULDN'T BE NICE

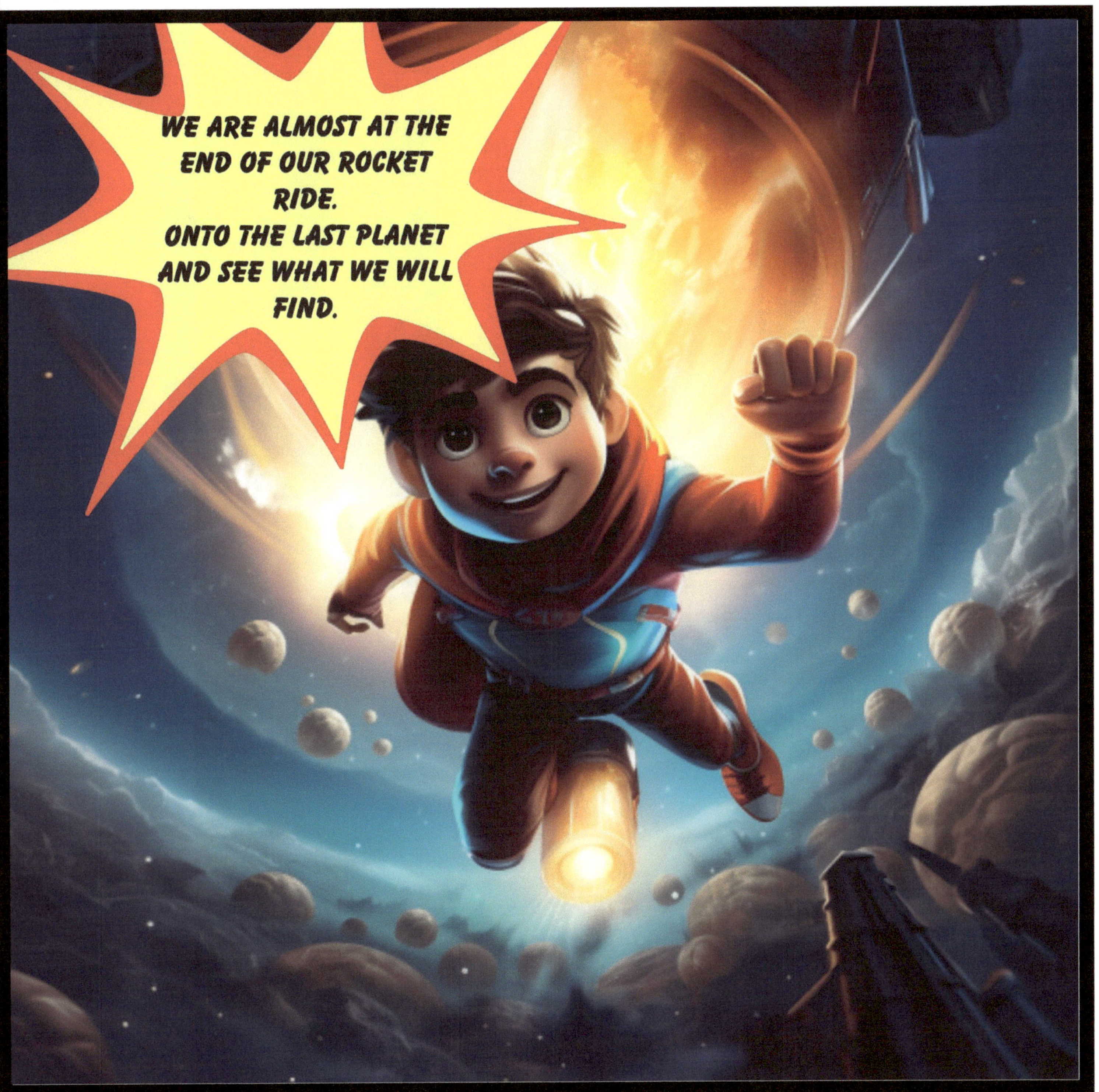

WE ARE ALMOST AT THE END OF OUR ROCKET RIDE.
ONTO THE LAST PLANET AND SEE WHAT WE WILL FIND.

# Neptune

FAST FACT
Uranus is four times wider than Earth
ANOTHER ICE GIANT AND THIS ONE IS CALLED NEPTUNE. WE'LL FLY ROUND IT'S FIVE RINGS AND I'LL TAKE YOU BACK HOME SOON.

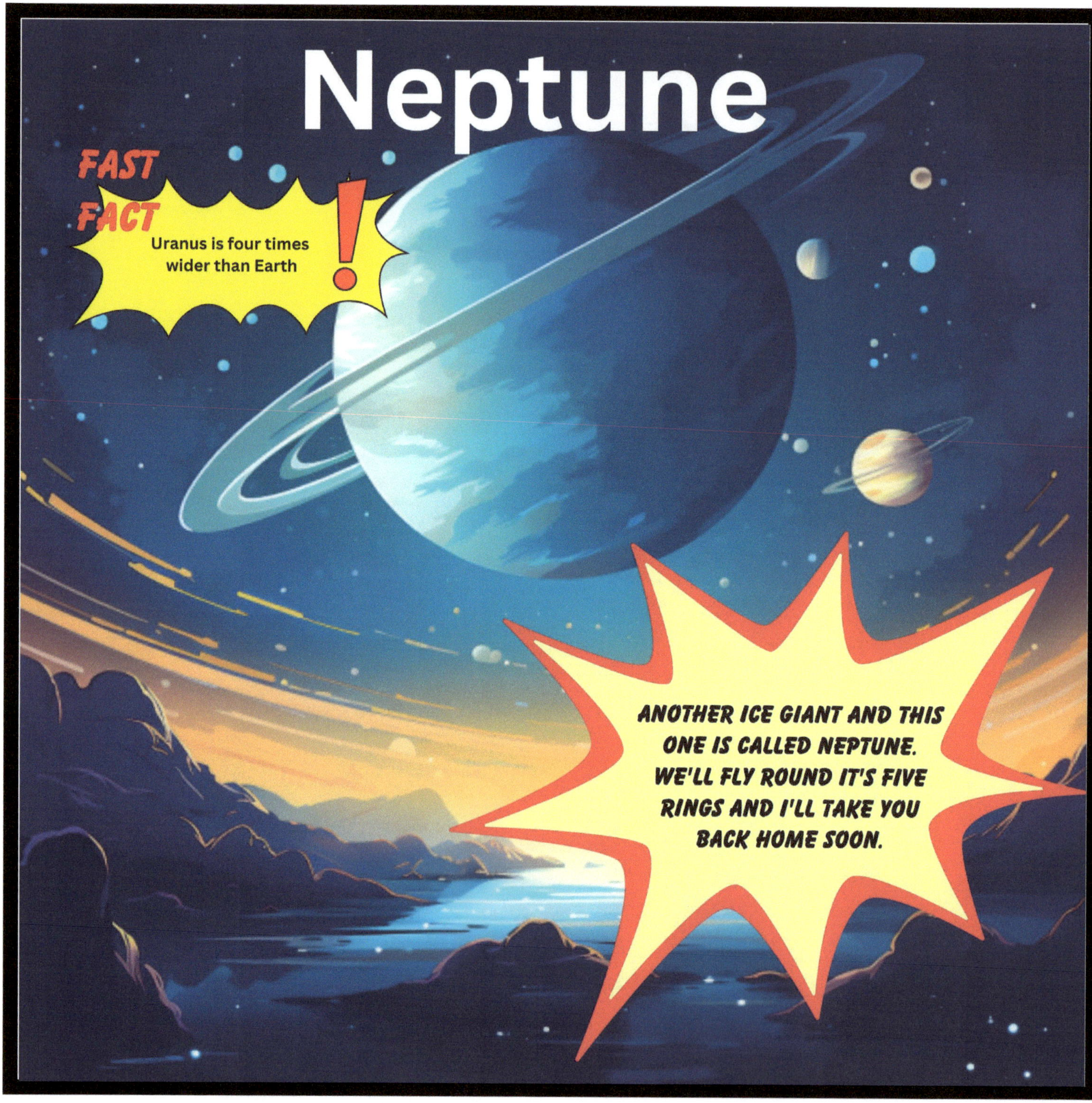

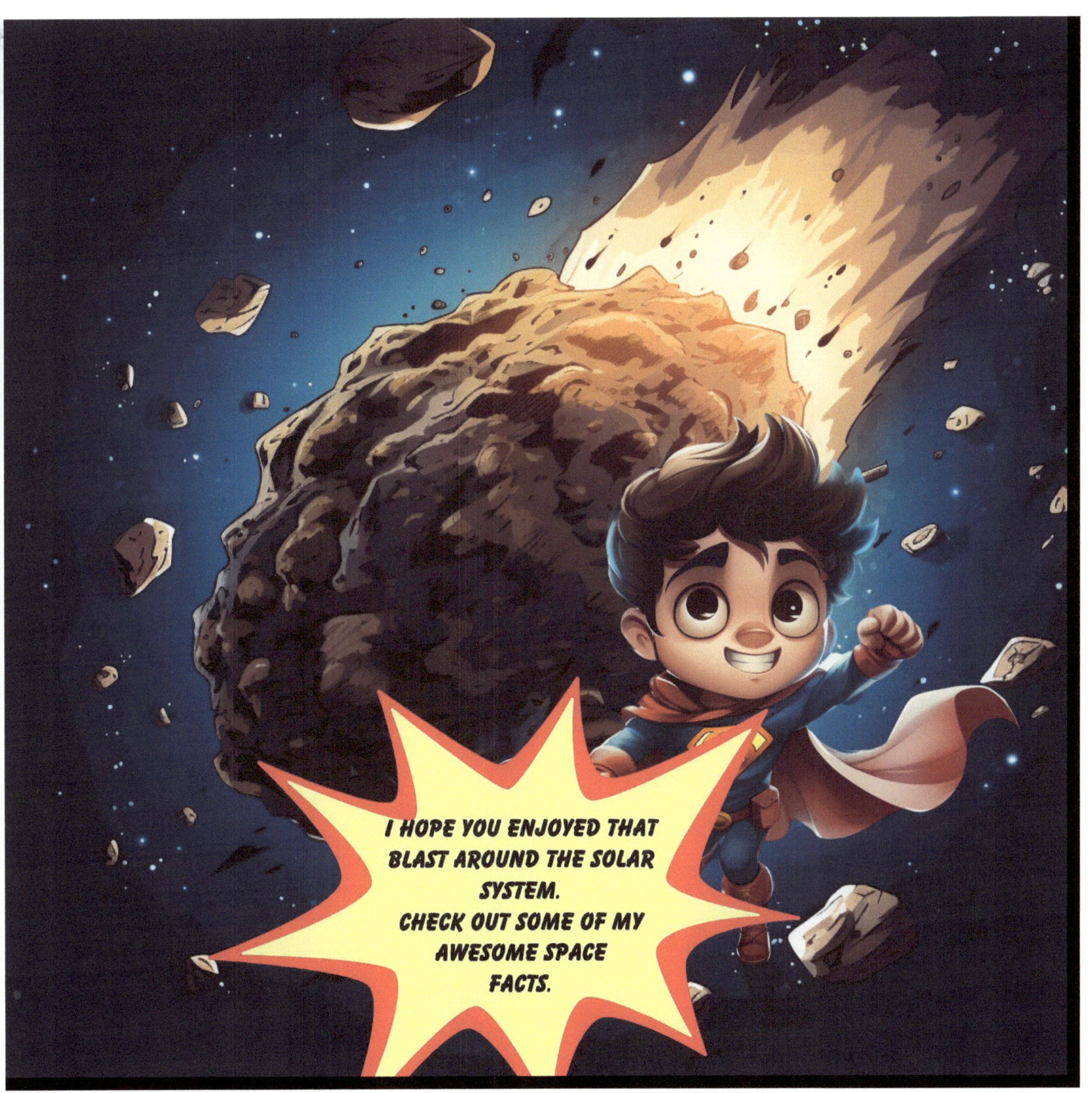
I HOPE YOU ENJOYED THAT BLAST AROUND THE SOLAR SYSTEM.
CHECK OUT SOME OF MY AWESOME SPACE FACTS.

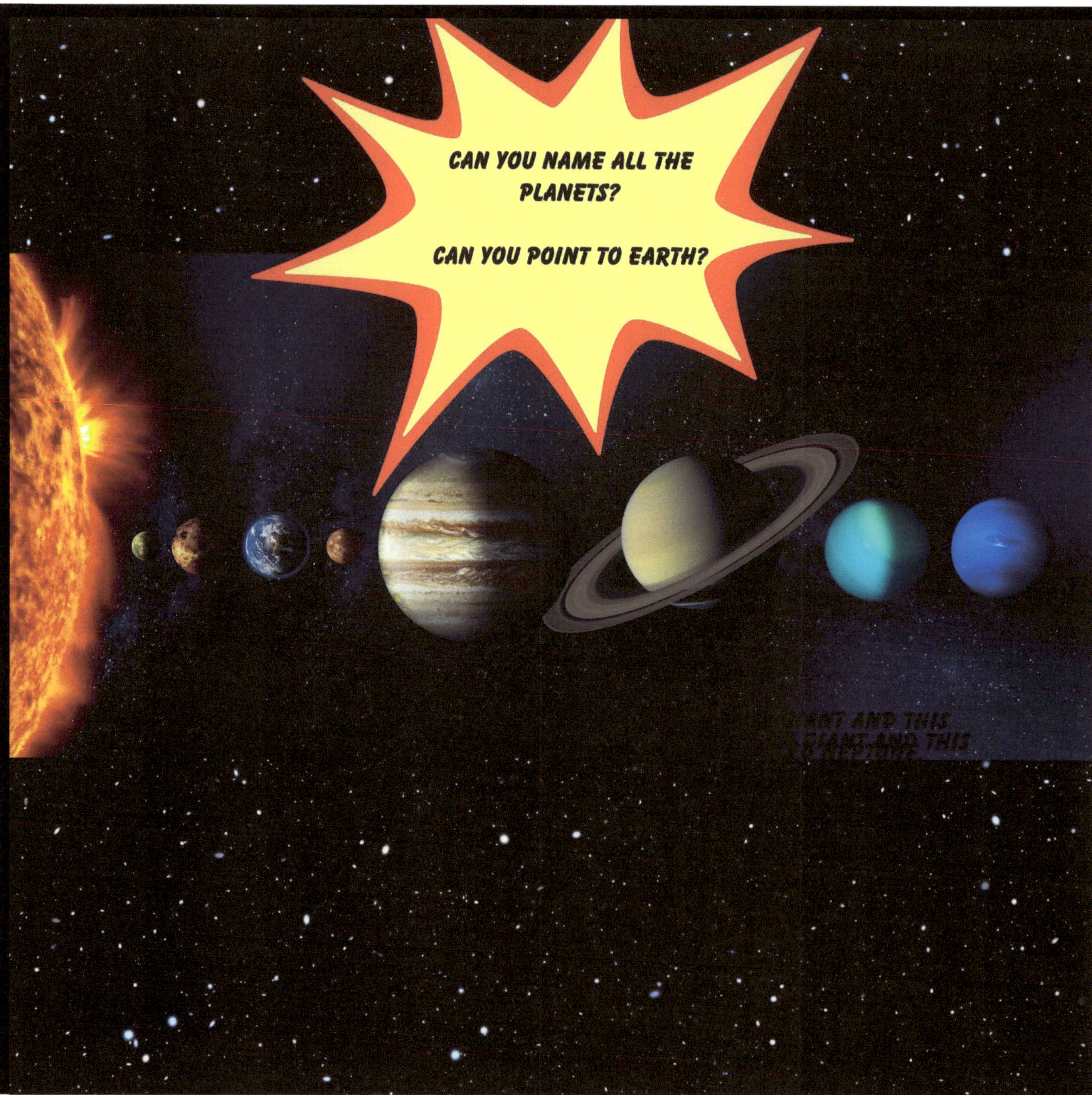

CAN YOU NAME ALL THE PLANETS?
CAN YOU POINT TO EARTH?

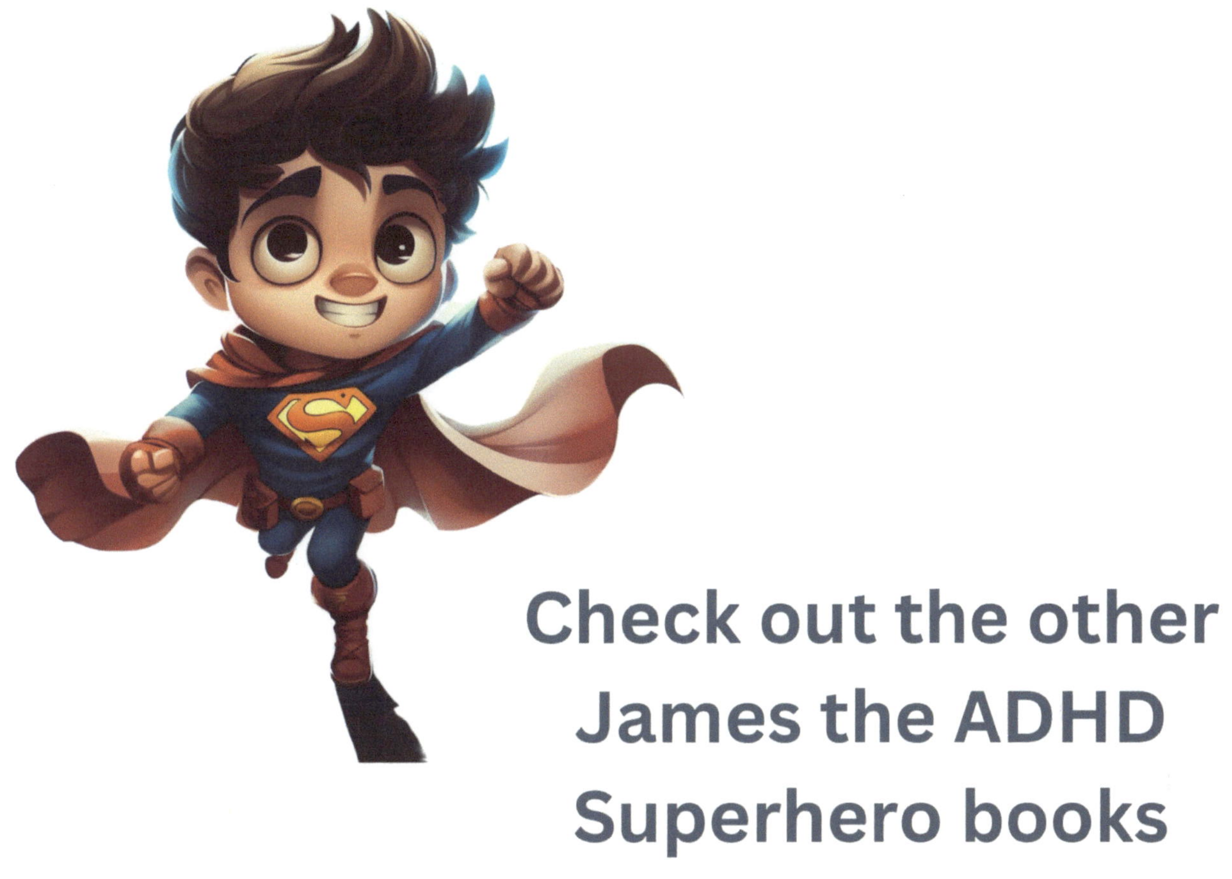

Check out the other James the ADHD Superhero books

# The End